HOW TO CURE CANCER NATURALLY FROM HOME INSPIRED BY DR. BARBARA O'NEILL

Discover proven natural and holistic methods to heal and cure cancer

Ben Hans

Table of Contents

CHAPTER ONE 4

   Introduction: The Power of Natural Healing 4

   History and Origins 4

   Philosophy and Principles 5

   Modalities and Practices 6

   Evidence and Controversy 7

CHAPTER TWO 9

   Understanding Cancer: Types, Causes, and Progression 9

   Types of Cancer 9

   Causes of Cancer 11

   Conclusion 14

CHAPTER THREE 15

   The Philosophy Behind Dr. Barbara's Herbal Approach 15

CHAPTER FOUR 18

   Preparing for Your Healing Journey: Mental and Physical Readiness 18

CHAPTER FIVE 22

   Key Herbs and Plants for Natural Cancer Treatment 22

CHAPTER SIX 26

   Implementing herbal therapies at home 26

CHAPTER SEVEN 30

Nutritional strategies	30
CHAPTER EIGHT	**34**
Making lifestyle adjustments	34
CHAPTER NINE	**38**
Overcoming challenges and staying motivated during cancer treatment	38
BONUS: SOME HERBAL REMEDIES TO KNOW	42
THE END	**76**

COPYRIGHT © 2023

All rights reserved. No part of this publication may be reproduced, distributed, or transmitted in any form or by any means, including photocopying, recording, or other electronic or mechanical methods, without the prior written permission of the publisher, except in the case of brief quotations embodied in critical reviews and certain other noncommercial uses permitted by copyright law.

CHAPTER ONE

Introduction: The Power of Natural Healing

Natural healing, often referred to as alternative or holistic medicine, encompasses a diverse array of therapeutic approaches that prioritize the body's innate ability to heal itself. It stands in contrast to conventional Western medicine, which typically relies on pharmaceuticals and surgical interventions to treat symptoms of illness or disease. The foundation of natural healing lies in ancient traditions and indigenous practices that have been passed down through generations, evolving and adapting over time.

At its core, natural healing acknowledges the interconnectedness of mind, body, and spirit, recognizing that imbalances in one aspect can manifest as physical or emotional ailments. It emphasizes the importance of addressing underlying root causes rather than merely alleviating symptoms, aiming for comprehensive wellness rather than simply the absence of disease.

History and Origins

The history of natural healing is as rich and diverse as the cultures from which it emerged. Ancient civilizations such as those in China, India, Egypt, and Greece developed sophisticated systems of medicine based on observations of the natural world and the body's inner workings. These early healers recognized the role of diet, lifestyle, and environment in maintaining health and sought to restore balance through methods such as herbal remedies, acupuncture, yoga, and meditation.

In traditional Chinese medicine (TCM), for example, illness is seen as an imbalance of the body's vital energy, or qi (pronounced "chee"). Practitioners use techniques such as acupuncture, herbal medicine, and qigong to promote the flow of qi and restore harmony within the body. Similarly, Ayurveda, India's ancient healing system, focuses on balancing the three doshas—vata, pitta, and kapha—to maintain health and prevent disease through practices like dietary adjustments, herbal medicine, and yoga.

Philosophy and Principles

Central to natural healing is a philosophy rooted in the belief that the body possesses an innate intelligence and capacity for self-repair. This belief aligns with the concept of vitalism, which posits that living organisms are governed by a vital force or energy that distinguishes them from inanimate matter. From this perspective, health is not merely the absence of disease but a state of dynamic equilibrium and vitality.

The principles of natural healing emphasize the interconnectedness of all aspects of health, including physical, mental, emotional, and spiritual well-being. Rather than viewing symptoms in isolation, practitioners seek to understand the underlying causes of illness, which may stem from factors such as poor nutrition, stress, environmental toxins, or unresolved emotional traumas.

Modalities and Practices

Natural healing encompasses a diverse range of modalities and practices, each offering unique approaches to restoring balance and promoting wellness. Some of the most widely recognized modalities include:

1. **Herbal Medicine:** Herbal remedies have been used for millennia to support health and treat a wide range of ailments. Plants contain a wealth of bioactive compounds with medicinal properties, and herbalists carefully select and combine herbs to address specific health concerns.

2. **Nutritional Therapy:** Food is considered not only sustenance but also medicine in natural healing traditions. Nutritional therapy focuses on optimizing diet and lifestyle to support overall health and prevent disease. This may involve personalized dietary recommendations, supplementation, and lifestyle modifications.

3. **Mind-Body Medicine:** The mind-body connection plays a central role in natural healing, with practices such as meditation, yoga, tai chi, and mindfulness-based stress reduction being widely utilized to promote relaxation, reduce stress, and enhance overall well-being.

4. **Energy Medicine:** Energy-based therapies work with the body's subtle energy systems to restore balance and facilitate healing. Techniques such as acupuncture, acupressure, reiki, and therapeutic touch are based on the premise that disruptions in the body's energy flow can lead to illness and can be corrected through various interventions.

5. **Manual Therapies:** Hands-on therapies such as chiropractic, osteopathy, massage therapy, and craniosacral therapy focus on manipulating the body's structure to relieve pain, improve mobility, and enhance overall function.

Evidence and Controversy

Despite the growing popularity of natural healing approaches, they have often been met with skepticism and controversy within the medical establishment. Critics argue that many alternative therapies lack rigorous scientific evidence to support their efficacy and safety, and caution against relying on them as primary treatment modalities for serious or life-threatening conditions.

However, proponents of natural healing point to a growing body of research that supports the effectiveness of various modalities, particularly in the realm of chronic disease management, pain relief, and stress reduction. Moreover, they emphasize the importance of individualized care and the integration of complementary therapies with conventional medicine to achieve optimal outcomes for patients.

Conclusion

Natural healing offers a holistic approach to health and wellness that honors the body's innate capacity for healing and regeneration. Rooted in ancient traditions and informed by modern science, it encompasses a diverse array of modalities and practices that address the interconnectedness of mind, body, and spirit. While controversy and skepticism persist, the growing body of evidence supporting the efficacy of natural healing approaches highlights their potential to complement conventional medicine and empower individuals to take an active role in their health and well-being.

CHAPTER TWO

Understanding Cancer: Types, Causes, and Progression

Cancer is a complex and multifaceted group of diseases characterized by the uncontrolled growth and spread of abnormal cells. It is one of the leading causes of morbidity and mortality worldwide, posing significant challenges to public health systems and affecting millions of individuals and families each year. To fully comprehend cancer, it's crucial to delve into its various types, understand its underlying causes, and grasp its progression within the body.

Types of Cancer

Cancer can arise in virtually any tissue or organ of the body, giving rise to a diverse range of cancer types. Some of the most common forms of cancer include:

1. **Carcinomas:** These cancers originate in the epithelial cells that line the surfaces and cavities of organs, such as the skin, lungs, breast, prostate, and colon. Carcinomas account for the majority of cancer cases and can spread to nearby tissues and organs (invasive carcinoma) or remain localized (in situ carcinoma).

2. **Sarcomas:** Sarcomas develop in the connective tissues, including bones, muscles, cartilage, and blood vessels.

Examples of sarcomas include osteosarcoma (bone cancer), leiomyosarcoma (smooth muscle cancer), and liposarcoma (fat tissue cancer).

3. **Leukemias:** Leukemias are cancers of the blood-forming tissues, such as the bone marrow and lymphatic system. They involve the abnormal proliferation of white blood cells and can be classified into four main types: acute lymphoblastic leukemia (ALL), acute myeloid leukemia (AML), chronic lymphocytic leukemia (CLL), and chronic myeloid leukemia (CML).

4. **Lymphomas:** Lymphomas affect the lymphatic system, which includes lymph nodes, spleen, thymus, and bone marrow. They can be categorized as Hodgkin lymphoma or non-Hodgkin lymphoma, depending on the specific type of lymphocyte affected and other histological characteristics.

5. **Central Nervous System (CNS) Tumors:** These tumors arise in the brain or spinal cord and can be benign (non-cancerous) or malignant (cancerous). Examples include gliomas, meningiomas, and medulloblastomas.

These categories represent broad classifications, and there are numerous subtypes and variations of cancer within each group, each with its own distinct characteristics and treatment approaches.

Causes of Cancer

The development of cancer is a complex and multifactorial process influenced by a combination of genetic, environmental, and lifestyle factors. While the exact causes of many cancers remain elusive, researchers have identified several key factors that contribute to cancer development:

1. **Genetic Mutations:** Mutations in the DNA of cells can disrupt normal cellular functions, leading to uncontrolled growth and proliferation. These mutations can be inherited (germline mutations) or acquired during a person's lifetime (somatic mutations) due to exposure to carcinogens, radiation, or errors in DNA replication.

2. **Environmental Exposures:** Exposure to carcinogenic substances in the environment, such as tobacco smoke, asbestos, ultraviolet (UV) radiation, air pollutants, and certain chemicals, can increase the risk of developing cancer. These substances can damage DNA and trigger cellular changes that promote cancer formation.

3. **Lifestyle Factors:** Certain lifestyle choices, such as tobacco use, poor diet, lack of physical activity, excessive alcohol consumption, and obesity, are associated with an increased risk of cancer. These factors can contribute to chronic inflammation, oxidative stress, and hormonal imbalances that promote tumor growth and progression.

4. **Viral Infections:** Some cancers are caused by viral infections, such as human papillomavirus (HPV), hepatitis B virus (HBV), hepatitis C virus (HCV), Epstein-Barr virus (EBV), and human immunodeficiency virus (HIV). These viruses can disrupt normal cellular processes and trigger malignant transformation.

5. **Heredity:** Inherited genetic mutations can predispose individuals to certain types of cancer, such as breast cancer (BRCA1 and BRCA2 mutations), colorectal cancer (Lynch syndrome), and ovarian cancer (BRCA1 and BRCA2 mutations). While hereditary cancers represent a small percentage of overall cancer cases, they tend to occur at younger ages and may have a strong familial pattern.

Understanding the interplay between these factors is essential for elucidating the mechanisms underlying cancer development and identifying strategies for prevention and early detection.

Progression of Cancer

The progression of cancer involves a series of complex steps, beginning with the initiation of abnormal cellular growth and culminating in the formation of a malignant tumor and metastasis to distant sites. This process can be broadly categorized into several stages:

1. **Initiation:** Initiation occurs when normal cells undergo genetic mutations or epigenetic changes that confer a growth advantage and resistance to normal regulatory mechanisms. These alterations may be triggered by carcinogens, radiation, viruses, or genetic predisposition.

2. **Promotion:** Promotion involves the clonal expansion of initiated cells in response to proliferative signals from the tumor microenvironment. This stage is characterized by the accumulation of additional genetic alterations that further drive tumor growth and progression.

3. **Progression:** Progression marks the transition from pre-malignant lesions to invasive cancer, characterized by the acquisition of invasive and metastatic capabilities. Tumor cells may undergo epithelial-mesenchymal transition (EMT), enabling them to invade surrounding tissues, penetrate blood and lymphatic vessels, and disseminate to distant organs.

4. **Metastasis:** Metastasis is the spread of cancer cells from the primary tumor to distant sites in the body, facilitated by tumor cell intravasation, extravasation, and colonization. Metastatic dissemination is a complex and inefficient process influenced by interactions between tumor cells and the host microenvironment.

5. **Angiogenesis:** Angiogenesis, the formation of new blood vessels, plays a critical role in tumor growth and metastasis by supplying oxygen and nutrients to proliferating cancer cells. Tumor angiogenesis is driven by a complex interplay of pro-angiogenic and anti-angiogenic factors produced by tumor cells, stromal cells, and immune cells.

Understanding the dynamic nature of cancer progression is essential for developing targeted therapies that disrupt key molecular pathways involved in tumor growth, metastasis, and angiogenesis.

Conclusion

Cancer is a heterogeneous group of diseases characterized by abnormal cellular growth and proliferation. It arises from a complex interplay of genetic, environmental, and lifestyle factors and progresses through a series of stages, culminating in the formation of malignant tumors and metastasis to distant sites. By understanding the various types of cancer, their underlying causes, and the mechanisms of cancer progression, researchers and clinicians can develop more effective strategies for prevention, early detection, and treatment, ultimately improving outcomes for patients affected by this devastating disease.

CHAPTER THREE

The Philosophy Behind Dr. Barbara's Herbal Approach

Dr. Barbara's herbal approach to health and wellness is grounded in a holistic philosophy that emphasizes the interconnectedness of the body, mind, and spirit. Drawing upon principles from traditional herbal medicine, naturopathy, and holistic health practices, Dr. Barbara's approach seeks to restore balance and harmony within the body, supporting its innate healing capabilities and promoting overall well-being. At the core of Dr. Barbara's philosophy are several key principles that guide her herbal practice:

1. Wholistic Wellness: Dr. Barbara views health as a dynamic state of wholeness encompassing physical, mental, emotional, and spiritual aspects. Rather than focusing solely on treating symptoms or isolated conditions, she takes a comprehensive approach that addresses the underlying root causes of imbalance. By considering the interconnectedness of all aspects of health, Dr. Barbara aims to support the body's natural ability to heal itself and maintain equilibrium.

2. Vitalism: Central to Dr. Barbara's herbal philosophy is the concept of vitalism, which posits that living organisms possess an inherent life force or energy that animates and sustains them. According to this worldview, health is not merely the absence of disease but a state of vibrant vitality and resilience. Dr. Barbara believes that herbal medicine works in harmony with the body's vital force, nourishing and strengthening it to promote optimal health and vitality.

3. Nature as Healer: Nature serves as a potent source of healing and restoration in Dr. Barbara's herbal approach. She harnesses the therapeutic power of plants, herbs, and botanical remedies that have been used for centuries in traditional healing systems around the world. By honoring the wisdom of nature and respecting the inherent intelligence of plants, Dr. Barbara seeks to provide gentle yet effective remedies that support the body's natural healing processes.

4. Individualized Care: Recognizing that each person is unique, Dr. Barbara emphasizes the importance of individualized care in her herbal practice. She takes into account each individual's constitution, health history, lifestyle, and specific health concerns when formulating personalized herbal remedies. By tailoring her approach to the unique needs of each client, Dr. Barbara seeks to optimize therapeutic outcomes and empower individuals to take an active role in their health and wellness.

5. Prevention and Maintenance: In addition to addressing acute health issues, Dr. Barbara's herbal approach prioritizes prevention and maintenance of health. She advocates for proactive self-care practices, such as balanced nutrition, regular exercise, stress management, and adequate rest, as foundational pillars of wellness. By fostering healthy habits and lifestyle choices, Dr. Barbara aims to prevent illness and promote long-term vitality and resilience.

6. Empowerment and Education: Dr. Barbara believes in empowering individuals to become active participants in their own healing journey. She provides education and guidance to her clients, empowering them with knowledge about herbal medicine, nutrition, lifestyle modifications, and self-care practices. By fostering a deeper understanding of their bodies and health, Dr. Barbara empowers her clients to make informed choices and take ownership of their well-being.

In summary, Dr. Barbara's herbal approach is rooted in a holistic philosophy that recognizes the interconnectedness of body, mind, and spirit. By embracing principles of wholistic wellness, vitalism, nature as healer, individualized care, prevention and maintenance, and empowerment and education, Dr. Barbara seeks to support her clients in achieving optimal health, vitality, and well-being through the transformative power of herbal medicine.

CHAPTER FOUR

Preparing for Your Healing Journey: Mental and Physical Readiness

Embarking on a healing journey, whether it involves conventional medical treatment, alternative therapies, or a combination of both, requires careful preparation and readiness on both mental and physical levels. This preparatory phase sets the foundation for successful outcomes, facilitating the body's innate healing processes and optimizing the effectiveness of therapeutic interventions. In this discussion, we will explore the importance of mental and physical readiness in preparing for a healing journey and provide practical strategies for cultivating readiness in both domains.

Mental Readiness

Mental readiness encompasses a mindset characterized by openness, resilience, and commitment to the healing process. Cultivating mental readiness involves:

1. Acceptance and Openness: Embracing a mindset of acceptance and openness to the healing journey is essential. This involves acknowledging your current health status, understanding the challenges ahead, and being receptive to new perspectives, treatment modalities, and lifestyle changes.

2. Positive Attitude: Maintaining a positive attitude and optimistic outlook can have a profound impact on healing outcomes. Cultivate gratitude, optimism, and resilience in the face of challenges, and focus on the potential for growth, transformation, and healing.

3. Emotional Resilience: Building emotional resilience involves developing coping strategies to manage stress, anxiety, fear, and other emotions that may arise during the healing process. Practice mindfulness, relaxation techniques, deep breathing, and self-care activities to promote emotional well-being and balance.

4. Trust and Faith: Trusting in your healthcare providers, treatment plan, and the healing process itself is crucial. Cultivate faith in your body's innate ability to heal, as well as in the expertise of your healthcare team and the efficacy of chosen therapies.

5. Commitment to Self-Care: Prioritize self-care practices that nourish your mind, body, and spirit. This may include engaging in activities you enjoy, spending time in nature, nurturing supportive relationships, practicing gratitude, and setting boundaries to protect your well-being.

Physical Readiness

Physical readiness involves preparing your body to undergo the healing process and optimizing its capacity for recovery. Key aspects of physical readiness include:

1. Nutrition: Adopting a balanced and nutritious diet is fundamental to supporting your body's healing processes. Focus on consuming whole, nutrient-dense foods that provide essential vitamins, minerals, antioxidants, and phytonutrients. Limit processed foods, refined sugars, and inflammatory substances that can impede healing.

2. Exercise and Movement: Regular physical activity is essential for promoting circulation, mobility, strength, and overall well-being. Incorporate gentle exercises, such as walking, yoga, tai chi, or swimming, into your daily routine to support your body's healing and recovery.

3. Sleep and Rest: Adequate sleep and rest are critical for cellular repair, immune function, and overall health. Prioritize quality sleep by establishing a consistent sleep schedule, creating a relaxing bedtime routine, and optimizing your sleep environment for restorative rest.

4. Hydration: Proper hydration is essential for maintaining cellular function, detoxification, and overall health. Drink plenty of water throughout the day to stay hydrated and support your body's natural healing processes.

5. Medication Management: If you are taking medications or undergoing medical treatments, ensure that you follow your healthcare provider's recommendations carefully. Adhere to prescribed medication regimens, attend follow-up appointments, and communicate openly with your healthcare team about any concerns or side effects.

Conclusion

Preparing for a healing journey requires a holistic approach that addresses both mental and physical aspects of readiness. By cultivating acceptance, positivity, resilience, and trust on a mental level, and prioritizing nutrition, exercise, sleep, hydration, and medication management on a physical level, you can optimize your body's capacity for healing and promote positive outcomes. Remember that healing is a journey, and progress may unfold gradually over time. Stay patient, compassionate, and committed to your well-being, and trust in the process of healing and transformation.

CHAPTER FIVE

Key Herbs and Plants for Natural Cancer Treatment

Natural cancer treatment approaches often incorporate the use of herbs and plants that have been traditionally used for their anti-cancer properties. While it's essential to approach natural treatments with caution and consult with healthcare professionals, several herbs and plants have shown promising anti-cancer effects in preclinical studies and anecdotal evidence. Here are some key herbs and plants commonly used in natural cancer treatment:

1. Turmeric (Curcuma longa): Turmeric contains curcumin, a compound with potent anti-inflammatory and antioxidant properties. Research suggests that curcumin may inhibit cancer cell proliferation, induce apoptosis (cell death), and suppress tumor growth in various types of cancer, including breast, prostate, colorectal, and pancreatic cancer.

2. Green Tea (Camellia sinensis): Green tea is rich in polyphenols, particularly epigallocatechin gallate (EGCG), which has been studied for its anti-cancer effects. EGCG has been shown to inhibit cancer cell growth, induce apoptosis, and inhibit angiogenesis (the formation of new blood vessels that support tumor growth) in several types of cancer, including breast, prostate, lung, and colorectal cancer.

3. Reishi Mushroom (Ganoderma lucidum): Reishi mushroom, also known as Lingzhi, is revered in traditional Chinese medicine for its immune-modulating and anti-cancer properties. Studies suggest that reishi mushroom extracts may inhibit cancer cell proliferation, enhance immune function, and induce apoptosis in various types of cancer, including lung, breast, prostate, and colorectal cancer.

4. Ginger (Zingiber officinale): Ginger contains bioactive compounds such as gingerol, which has demonstrated anti-inflammatory, antioxidant, and anti-cancer effects. Research suggests that ginger may inhibit cancer cell growth, induce apoptosis, and suppress tumor angiogenesis in several types of cancer, including ovarian, colorectal, and pancreatic cancer.

5. Garlic (Allium sativum): Garlic is rich in organosulfur compounds, such as allicin, which exhibit potent anti-cancer properties. Studies suggest that garlic may inhibit cancer cell proliferation, induce apoptosis, and inhibit tumor growth and metastasis in various types of cancer, including breast, lung, and colorectal cancer.

6. Astragalus (Astragalus membranaceus): Astragalus is an herb used in traditional Chinese medicine for its immune-boosting and anti-cancer properties. Research suggests that astragalus extracts may enhance immune function, inhibit cancer cell proliferation, and suppress tumor growth in several types of cancer, including lung, breast, and liver cancer.

7. Milk Thistle (Silybum marianum): Milk thistle contains a flavonoid complex known as silymarin, which has antioxidant and anti-inflammatory properties. Silymarin has been studied for its potential anti-cancer effects and may inhibit cancer cell growth, induce apoptosis, and enhance chemotherapy efficacy in certain types of cancer, including prostate, breast, and liver cancer.

8. Cat's Claw (Uncaria tomentosa): Cat's claw is a woody vine native to the Amazon rainforest, traditionally used in indigenous medicine for its anti-inflammatory and immune-modulating properties. Research suggests that cat's claw extracts may inhibit cancer cell proliferation, induce apoptosis, and enhance immune function in various types of cancer, including breast, prostate, and colorectal cancer.

9. Essiac Tea (Blend of Burdock Root, Sheep Sorrel, Slippery Elm Bark, and Indian Rhubarb Root): Essiac tea is a herbal blend originally developed by Ojibwa Native Americans and later popularized as a natural cancer remedy. While clinical evidence is limited, some studies and anecdotal reports suggest that Essiac tea may have anti-cancer effects and support immune function in cancer patients.

10. Graviola (Annona muricata): Graviola, also known as soursop, is a tropical fruit tree whose leaves, fruit, and seeds have been used in traditional medicine for their potential anti-cancer properties. Some laboratory studies have shown that graviola extracts may inhibit cancer cell growth and induce apoptosis in various types of cancer, including breast, prostate, and pancreatic cancer.

While these herbs and plants show promise in preclinical studies and traditional use, it's essential to approach natural cancer treatments with caution and consult with healthcare professionals, especially if you are undergoing conventional cancer treatment. Natural remedies should complement, not replace, standard medical care, and individual responses to herbs and plants may vary. Additionally, some herbs may interact with medications or have contraindications for certain health conditions. Always consult with a qualified healthcare practitioner before incorporating herbs or supplements into your cancer treatment regimen.

CHAPTER SIX

Implementing herbal therapies at home

Implementing herbal therapies at home can be a rewarding and empowering way to support your health and well-being. Whether you're seeking to address specific health concerns, boost your immune system, or promote overall vitality, integrating herbal remedies into your daily routine can offer numerous benefits. Here are some practical steps to help you get started with implementing herbal therapies at home:

1. Educate Yourself: Start by educating yourself about different herbs, their properties, and potential therapeutic uses. There are many resources available, including books, online articles, and reputable websites dedicated to herbal medicine. Consider taking courses or workshops on herbalism to deepen your knowledge and understanding of herbal therapies.

2. Identify Your Health Goals: Determine your specific health goals and areas of concern that you would like to address with herbal therapies. Whether you're looking to support digestion, reduce stress, improve sleep, or boost immunity, there are herbs available to suit your needs.

3. Consult with a Qualified Herbalist: If you're new to herbal medicine or have complex health issues, consider consulting with a qualified herbalist or holistic healthcare practitioner. A professional herbalist can offer personalized guidance and recommendations based on your individual health history, constitution, and goals.

4. Start Slowly: Begin by incorporating one or two herbal remedies into your routine and gradually expand as you become more comfortable and familiar with their effects. Start with simple preparations, such as herbal teas, tinctures, or capsules, and experiment with different herbs to find what works best for you.

5. Choose High-Quality Herbs: Select high-quality herbs from reputable sources to ensure purity, potency, and safety. Look for organic, sustainably harvested herbs whenever possible, and avoid herbs that may be contaminated with pesticides, heavy metals, or other toxins.

6. Experiment with Herbal Preparations: Explore different herbal preparations and methods of administration to find what works best for you. Herbal teas, tinctures, capsules, infused oils, salves, and poultices are just a few examples of herbal remedies that can be easily prepared at home.

7. Keep a Journal: Keep a journal to track your experiences with different herbs and herbal remedies. Note any changes in your symptoms, mood, energy levels, or overall well-being, as well as any side effects or adverse reactions. This will help you identify which herbs are most effective for your individual needs.

8. Practice Consistency: Consistency is key when it comes to herbal therapies. Incorporate herbal remedies into your daily routine and make them a regular part of your self-care regimen. Consistent use over time can yield cumulative benefits and support long-term health and wellness.

9. Monitor Your Progress: Pay attention to how your body responds to herbal therapies and make adjustments as needed. If you're not experiencing the desired effects, consider trying different herbs or adjusting your dosage or frequency of use. Be patient and give your body time to respond to herbal treatments.

10. Listen to Your Body: Listen to your body's cues and intuition when using herbal remedies. If something doesn't feel right or if you experience any adverse reactions, discontinue use and consult with a healthcare professional. Trust your instincts and honor your body's wisdom throughout your healing journey.

By following these steps and integrating herbal therapies into your daily life with care and intention, you can harness the healing power of plants to support your health and well-being naturally. Remember that herbal medicine is a complementary approach that works best when combined with other healthy lifestyle practices, such as balanced nutrition, regular exercise, stress management, and adequate rest. As always, consult with a healthcare professional before starting any new herbal remedies, especially if you have underlying health conditions or are taking medications.

CHAPTER SEVEN

Nutritional strategies

Nutritional strategies play a crucial role in supporting cancer healing and overall well-being. A balanced and nutrient-rich diet can help strengthen the immune system, support cellular repair and regeneration, reduce inflammation, and promote overall health during cancer treatment and recovery. Here are some key nutritional strategies to consider:

1. Emphasize Whole Foods:

- Focus on consuming a variety of whole, nutrient-dense foods, including fruits, vegetables, whole grains, legumes, nuts, seeds, and lean proteins. These foods provide essential vitamins, minerals, antioxidants, and phytonutrients that support immune function and cellular health.

2. Prioritize Plant-Based Foods:

- Plant-based foods are rich in phytonutrients and antioxidants that can help protect cells from damage and reduce the risk of chronic diseases, including cancer. Aim to include a wide variety of colorful fruits and vegetables in your diet, such as leafy greens, berries, citrus fruits, cruciferous vegetables, and colorful peppers.

3. Include Healthy Fats:

- Incorporate healthy fats into your diet from sources such as avocados, olive oil, nuts, seeds, and fatty fish (e.g., salmon, mackerel, sardines). These fats provide essential omega-3 fatty acids, which have anti-inflammatory properties and support brain health, cardiovascular health, and immune function.

4. Opt for Lean Proteins:

- Choose lean sources of protein, such as poultry, fish, tofu, tempeh, legumes, and low-fat dairy products. Protein is essential for tissue repair and muscle maintenance, especially during cancer treatment and recovery.

5. Limit Processed and Red Meat:

- Limit consumption of processed meats, such as bacon, sausage, deli meats, and hot dogs, as well as red meats like beef, pork, and lamb. These meats are high in saturated fat and may contain carcinogenic compounds that can increase the risk of cancer.

6. Minimize Added Sugars and Refined Carbohydrates:

- Reduce your intake of added sugars, sugary beverages, refined grains, and processed snacks, which can contribute to inflammation, insulin resistance, and weight gain. Instead, choose whole grains (e.g., brown rice, quinoa, oats), fruits, and vegetables as primary sources of carbohydrates.

7. Stay Hydrated:

- Drink plenty of water throughout the day to stay hydrated and support cellular function, detoxification, and overall health. Aim for at least 8-10 cups of water per day, and consider incorporating hydrating foods like cucumbers, watermelon, and citrus fruits into your diet.

8. Focus on Anti-Inflammatory Foods:

- Include anti-inflammatory foods in your diet, such as turmeric, ginger, garlic, onions, berries, cherries, leafy greens, and fatty fish. These foods contain compounds that help reduce inflammation and may help alleviate symptoms associated with cancer and its treatment.

9. Consider Nutritional Supplements:

- Talk to your healthcare provider about incorporating nutritional supplements into your regimen, especially if you have specific nutrient deficiencies or difficulty meeting your nutritional needs through diet alone. Supplements such as vitamin D, omega-3 fatty acids, probiotics, and multivitamins may be beneficial for supporting overall health and immune function.

10. Practice Mindful Eating:

- Practice mindful eating by paying attention to hunger and fullness cues, eating slowly, and savoring each bite. Listen to your body's signals and choose foods that make you feel nourished, energized, and satisfied.

11. Seek Professional Guidance:

- Work with a registered dietitian or nutritionist who specializes in oncology nutrition to develop a personalized nutrition plan tailored to your specific needs, preferences, and treatment goals. A qualified professional can provide evidence-based guidance, support, and education to help you optimize your nutritional intake and support your cancer healing journey.

By incorporating these nutritional strategies into your daily routine and working closely with your healthcare team, you can support your body's healing process, enhance your overall well-being, and improve your quality of life during cancer treatment and recovery. Remember that nutrition is just one aspect of cancer care, and it's essential to take a comprehensive approach that addresses all aspects of health and wellness.

CHAPTER EIGHT

Making lifestyle adjustments

Making lifestyle adjustments can be a powerful way to enhance your healing process and support overall well-being, especially during times of illness or recovery from cancer treatment. By incorporating positive lifestyle habits into your daily routine, you can optimize your physical, mental, and emotional health, promote healing, and improve your quality of life. Here are some lifestyle adjustments to consider:

1. Prioritize Stress Management:

- Chronic stress can have a negative impact on the immune system and overall health. Prioritize stress management techniques such as deep breathing, meditation, yoga, tai chi, progressive muscle relaxation, mindfulness, and spending time in nature. Find activities that help you relax and unwind, and make them a regular part of your routine.

2. Get Regular Exercise:

- Physical activity has numerous benefits for both physical and mental health. Aim to incorporate regular exercise into your routine, focusing on activities that you enjoy and that are appropriate for your fitness level. Choose activities such as walking, swimming, cycling, yoga, or gentle strength training to improve circulation, strength, flexibility, and mood.

3. Maintain a Healthy Weight:

- Achieving and maintaining a healthy weight is important for overall health and well-being, especially during cancer treatment and recovery. Focus on adopting a balanced diet rich in whole foods and lean proteins, and aim to engage in regular physical activity to support weight management and overall health.

4. Prioritize Sleep Hygiene:

- Quality sleep is essential for healing and overall well-being. Practice good sleep hygiene habits, such as maintaining a consistent sleep schedule, creating a relaxing bedtime routine, avoiding stimulants like caffeine and electronics before bed, and ensuring your sleep environment is comfortable and conducive to restorative rest.

5. Foster Supportive Relationships:

- Cultivate supportive relationships with friends, family members, and healthcare providers who can offer emotional support, encouragement, and practical assistance during your healing journey. Share your feelings and experiences with trusted loved ones, and don't hesitate to ask for help when needed.

6. Engage in Meaningful Activities:

- Stay engaged in activities and hobbies that bring you joy, fulfillment, and a sense of purpose. Whether it's spending time with loved ones, pursuing creative interests, volunteering, or connecting with your community, engaging in meaningful activities can boost mood, reduce stress, and enhance overall well-being.

7. Practice Self-Care:

- Prioritize self-care activities that nourish your mind, body, and spirit. This may include practices such as journaling, spending time in nature, taking relaxing baths, practicing gratitude, engaging in creative expression, and setting boundaries to protect your well-being.

8. Limit Exposure to Toxins:

- Minimize exposure to environmental toxins and carcinogens by choosing natural, eco-friendly household products, avoiding tobacco smoke and other pollutants, eating organic foods whenever possible, and reducing consumption of processed foods and beverages with artificial additives.

9. Cultivate Resilience and Optimism:

- Cultivate resilience and optimism by focusing on positive thinking, finding meaning and purpose in your experiences, and practicing gratitude for the blessings in your life. Maintain a hopeful outlook and believe in your ability to overcome challenges and thrive, even in the face of adversity.

10. Stay Informed and Empowered:

- Take an active role in your healing process by staying informed about your condition, treatment options, and self-care strategies. Ask questions, seek out reliable information from reputable sources, and advocate for yourself as a partner in your healthcare journey.

By incorporating these lifestyle adjustments into your daily routine, you can create a supportive environment for healing, enhance your overall well-being, and optimize your quality of life during cancer treatment and recovery. Remember that small changes can have a big impact over time, so focus on making gradual, sustainable adjustments that align with your individual needs and preferences.

CHAPTER NINE

Overcoming challenges and staying motivated during cancer treatment

Overcoming challenges and staying motivated during cancer treatment or any healing journey can be difficult, but it's essential for maintaining resilience, hope, and a positive outlook. Here are some strategies to help you navigate challenges and stay motivated:

1. Build a Support System:

- Surround yourself with a supportive network of friends, family members, healthcare providers, and fellow survivors who can offer encouragement, empathy, and practical assistance. Lean on your support system during difficult times and share your feelings and experiences with trusted loved ones.

2. Set Realistic Goals:

- Break down your healing journey into manageable steps and set realistic, achievable goals for yourself. Celebrate small victories along the way and acknowledge your progress, no matter how incremental. Adjust your goals as needed to adapt to changing circumstances and priorities.

3. Practice Self-Compassion:

- Be gentle with yourself and practice self-compassion as you navigate challenges and setbacks. Treat yourself with kindness, understanding, and patience, and recognize that it's okay to feel a range of emotions, including sadness, anger, and frustration.

4. Stay Informed and Empowered:

- Educate yourself about your condition, treatment options, and self-care strategies so that you can make informed decisions and advocate for yourself as a partner in your healthcare journey. Stay engaged in your treatment plan and ask questions to clarify any concerns or uncertainties.

5. Focus on What You Can Control:

- Focus your energy on things that are within your control, such as your attitude, mindset, self-care practices, and daily habits. Let go of worrying about things beyond your control and channel your efforts into positive actions that promote healing and well-being.

6. Practice Mindfulness and Resilience:

- Cultivate mindfulness and resilience by staying present in the moment, practicing deep breathing, meditation, or relaxation techniques, and developing coping strategies to manage stress and anxiety. Draw upon your inner strength and resilience to navigate challenges with grace and courage.

7. Find Meaning and Purpose:

- Find meaning and purpose in your experiences by connecting with activities, hobbies, or causes that inspire you and bring you joy, fulfillment, and a sense of purpose. Focus on what truly matters to you and prioritize activities that align with your values and aspirations.

8. Seek Professional Support:

- Don't hesitate to seek professional support from therapists, counselors, or support groups who specialize in cancer care and survivorship. Professional support can provide valuable guidance, coping strategies, and emotional validation as you navigate the ups and downs of your healing journey.

9. Practice Gratitude and Positivity:

- Cultivate gratitude and positivity by focusing on the blessings and silver linings in your life, even during difficult times. Keep a gratitude journal, count your blessings, and surround yourself with uplifting messages, affirmations, and positive influences.

10. Celebrate Progress and Milestones:

- Celebrate your progress and milestones along the way, no matter how small they may seem. Recognize your resilience, strength, and courage in overcoming challenges and moving forward on your healing journey. Take time to acknowledge and honor your achievements.

Remember that overcoming challenges and staying motivated is a journey, and it's okay to have ups and downs along the way. Be patient with yourself, practice self-care, and draw upon your inner resources and support system to navigate challenges with resilience, hope, and determination. You are stronger and more resilient than you know, and you have the power to overcome obstacles and thrive, even in the face of adversity.

BONUS: SOME HERBAL REMEDIES TO KNOW

Bio Ferro Tonic:

Definition: Bio Ferro Tonic is a dietary supplement primarily composed of herbs and minerals. It's often marketed as a natural way to support overall health, particularly by promoting blood health and circulation.

Ingredients: Typical ingredients in Bio Ferro Tonic may include a blend of herbs such as burdock root, yellow dock root, sarsaparilla root, and cascara sagrada bark, along with minerals like iron and potassium phosphate.

How to Prepare: Bio Ferro Tonic usually comes in liquid form and is typically taken orally. It's important to follow the instructions on the product label for dosage and administration.

Dosage: The dosage can vary depending on the specific product and individual needs. It's crucial to consult with a healthcare professional or follow the recommended dosage on the product label to avoid potential side effects.

How to Use: Bio Ferro Tonic is often taken by adding the recommended dosage to water or juice and consuming it orally. It's important to shake the bottle well before use and store it according to the manufacturer's instructions.

Side Effects: While Bio Ferro Tonic is generally considered safe when used as directed, some individuals may experience side effects such as digestive discomfort, allergic reactions, or interactions with medications. It's essential to consult with a healthcare provider before starting any new supplement regimen, especially if you have underlying health conditions or are taking medications.

Bladderwrack:

Definition: Bladderwrack is a type of seaweed or marine algae commonly used in traditional medicine and as a dietary supplement. It's known for its potential health benefits, particularly related to thyroid health and weight management.

Ingredients: Bladderwrack contains various nutrients, including iodine, vitamins, minerals, and antioxidants. The primary active components are iodine and fucoidan, a type of carbohydrate found in brown seaweeds.

How to Prepare: Bladderwrack supplements are available in various forms, including capsules, powders, and liquid extracts. They can be taken orally with water or added to smoothies and other beverages.

Dosage: The appropriate dosage of bladderwrack can vary based on factors such as age, health status, and the specific product being used. It's essential to follow the recommended dosage on the product label or consult with a healthcare professional for personalized guidance.

How to Use: Bladderwrack supplements are typically taken orally, either with water or mixed into food or beverages. It's important to follow the instructions on the product label and avoid exceeding the recommended dosage.

Side Effects: While bladderwrack is generally considered safe for most people when used in moderation, excessive intake of iodine from bladderwrack supplements can cause thyroid dysfunction and other adverse effects. Individuals with thyroid disorders, iodine sensitivity, or certain medical conditions should exercise caution and consult with a healthcare provider before using bladderwrack supplements. Common side effects may include digestive upset, allergic reactions, or interactions with medications.

Blood Purifier:

Definition: Blood purifiers are herbal remedies or dietary supplements believed to cleanse or detoxify the blood, often promoting overall health and well-being. They are thought to support the body's natural detoxification processes and improve blood circulation.

Ingredients: Blood purifiers may contain a variety of herbs and botanical extracts known for their purported cleansing and detoxifying properties. Common ingredients include burdock root, red clover, dandelion root, and yellow dock root, among others.

How to Prepare: Blood purifiers are typically available in various forms, including capsules, tablets, powders, and liquid extracts. They are usually taken orally with water or juice, following the recommended dosage on the product label.

Dosage: The dosage of blood purifiers can vary depending on the specific product and individual needs. It's important to adhere to the recommended dosage on the product label or consult with a healthcare professional for personalized guidance.

How to Use: Blood purifiers are typically taken orally, either with water or mixed into beverages. They are often used as part of a detoxification regimen or to support overall health and vitality.

Side Effects: While blood purifiers are generally considered safe for most people when used as directed, some individuals may experience side effects such as digestive discomfort, allergic reactions, or interactions with medications. It's important to consult with a healthcare provider before starting any new supplement regimen, especially if you have underlying health conditions or are taking medications.

Blue Vervain:

Definition: Blue vervain, also known as Verbena hastata, is a perennial herb native to North America. It has been used in traditional medicine for centuries to treat various ailments, including anxiety, insomnia, and digestive issues.

Ingredients: Blue vervain contains several active compounds, including aucubin, verbenalin, and volatile oils. These compounds are believed to contribute to the herb's medicinal properties.

How to Prepare: Blue vervain is typically consumed as a tea or tincture. To make tea, dried blue vervain leaves and flowers are steeped in hot water for several minutes before being strained and consumed. Tinctures are prepared by steeping the herb in alcohol or vinegar to extract its active compounds.

Dosage: The appropriate dosage of blue vervain can vary depending on factors such as age, health status, and the specific preparation being used. It's important to follow the recommended dosage on the product label or consult with a qualified herbalist or healthcare professional for personalized guidance.

How to Use: Blue vervain tea or tincture is typically taken orally. It can be consumed on its own or mixed with honey or other herbal teas for added flavor.

Side Effects: While blue vervain is generally considered safe for most people when used in moderation, excessive intake may cause digestive upset or allergic reactions in some individuals. Pregnant or breastfeeding women should avoid blue vervain due to its potential to stimulate uterine contractions. As with any herbal remedy, it's important to consult with a healthcare provider before using blue vervain, especially if you have underlying health conditions or are taking medications.

Bromide Plus Powder:

Definition: Bromide Plus Powder is a dietary supplement formulated to support thyroid health and promote overall well-being. It typically contains a blend of herbs and minerals that are believed to have beneficial effects on thyroid function.

Ingredients: Bromide Plus Powder often contains a combination of herbs such as bladderwrack, sea moss, and burdock root, along with minerals like iodine and potassium phosphate. These ingredients are thought to support thyroid function and maintain optimal iodine levels in the body.

How to Prepare: Bromide Plus Powder is usually mixed with water or juice to create a drinkable solution. It's important to follow the instructions on the product label for dosage and preparation.

Dosage: The dosage of Bromide Plus Powder can vary depending on the specific product and individual needs. It's crucial to consult with a healthcare professional or follow the recommended dosage on the product label to avoid potential side effects.

How to Use: Bromide Plus Powder is typically taken orally by mixing the recommended dosage with water or juice. It's important to shake or stir the mixture well before consuming it to ensure even distribution of the ingredients.

Side Effects: While Bromide Plus Powder is generally considered safe when used as directed, some individuals may experience side effects such as digestive discomfort or allergic reactions to certain ingredients. It's essential to consult with a healthcare provider before starting any new supplement regimen, especially if you have underlying health conditions or are taking medications.

Bugleweed:

Definition: Bugleweed, also known as Lycopusvirginicus, is a perennial herb native to North America and Europe. It has been used in traditional medicine to treat various conditions, including hyperthyroidism, anxiety, and insomnia.

Ingredients: Bugleweed contains several active compounds, including lithospermic acid, phenolic acids, and flavonoids. These compounds are believed to contribute to the herb's medicinal properties, particularly its ability to regulate thyroid function.

How to Prepare: Bugleweed is commonly consumed as a tea or tincture. To make tea, dried bugleweed leaves and flowers are steeped in hot water for several minutes before being strained and consumed. Tinctures are prepared by steeping the herb in alcohol or vinegar to extract its active compounds.

Dosage: The appropriate dosage of bugleweed can vary depending on factors such as age, health status, and the specific preparation being used. It's important to follow the recommended dosage on the product label or consult with a qualified herbalist or healthcare professional for personalized guidance.

How to Use: Bugleweed tea or tincture is typically taken orally. It can be consumed on its own or mixed with honey or other herbal teas for added flavor.

Side Effects: While bugleweed is generally considered safe for most people when used in moderation, excessive intake may cause digestive upset or allergic reactions in some individuals. Pregnant or breastfeeding women should avoid bugleweed due to its potential to stimulate uterine contractions. As with any herbal remedy, it's important to consult with a healthcare provider before using bugleweed, especially if you have underlying health conditions or are taking medications.

Burdock:

Definition: Burdock, scientifically known as Arctium lappa, is a biennial plant native to Europe and Asia but now found worldwide. It's part of the Asteraceae family and has been used for centuries in traditional medicine and culinary practices.

Ingredients: Burdock contains various nutrients, including carbohydrates, fiber, vitamins (such as vitamin B6, folate, and vitamin C), and minerals (including potassium, magnesium, and manganese). It also contains active compounds such as polyphenols and volatile oils.

How to Prepare: Burdock can be prepared and consumed in various ways. The roots, leaves, and seeds are all utilized for different purposes. The root is commonly used in cooking, herbal teas, tinctures, and supplements, while the leaves and seeds are sometimes used in herbal preparations.

Dosage: The appropriate dosage of burdock root can vary depending on the specific form and intended use. For culinary purposes, there are no strict dosage guidelines, but for supplements or herbal remedies, it's essential to follow the recommended dosage on the product label or consult with a healthcare professional.

How to Use: Burdock root can be used in cooking by peeling, slicing, and adding it to soups, stews, stir-fries, or salads. It can also be brewed into a tea or used to make tinctures or extracts for medicinal purposes. Some people may also take burdock root supplements in capsule or powder form.

Side Effects: While burdock is generally considered safe for most people when consumed in moderate amounts, some individuals may experience allergic reactions or digestive upset. Additionally, burdock may interact with certain medications or have adverse effects in individuals with certain health conditions, such as diabetes or allergies to plants in the Asteraceae family. It's important to consult with a healthcare provider before using burdock, especially if you have underlying health conditions or are taking medications.

Cascara Sagrada:

Definition: Cascara Sagrada, scientifically known as Rhamnus purshiana, is a species of buckthorn native to western North America. It has been used traditionally as a laxative and to promote bowel regularity.

Ingredients: The primary active ingredients in cascara sagrada are anthraquinone glycosides, particularly cascarosides A and B. These compounds stimulate peristalsis in the colon, leading to increased bowel movements.

How to Prepare: Cascara sagrada is typically prepared as an herbal tea, tincture, or capsule. To make tea, dried cascara sagrada bark is steeped in hot water for several minutes before being strained and consumed. Tinctures are prepared by steeping the bark in alcohol to extract its active compounds.

Dosage: The appropriate dosage of cascara sagrada can vary depending on the specific preparation and intended use. It's important to follow the recommended dosage on the product label or consult with a healthcare professional for personalized guidance.

How to Use: Cascara sagrada tea or tincture is typically taken orally. It's important to start with a low dose and gradually increase if needed to avoid potential side effects such as cramping or diarrhea.

Side Effects: Cascara sagrada is considered safe for short-term use when used as directed. However, long-term or excessive use may lead to dependence, electrolyte imbalance, or dehydration. It may also interact with certain medications or have adverse effects in individuals with certain health conditions. It's important to use cascara sagrada under the guidance of a healthcare professional and to discontinue use if any adverse effects occur.

Cell Food:

Definition: Cell Food is a dietary supplement marketed as a highly oxygenating and alkalizing formula. It's claimed to support overall health and vitality by providing essential nutrients and oxygen to the cells.

Ingredients: The exact ingredients of Cell Food can vary depending on the brand, but it typically contains a proprietary blend of minerals, enzymes, electrolytes, and trace elements. Some common ingredients may include purified water, dissolved oxygen, seawater extract, and plant-based enzymes.

How to Prepare: Cell Food is usually available in liquid form and is typically taken orally. It can be consumed directly or diluted in water or juice before consumption.

Dosage: The dosage of Cell Food can vary depending on the specific product and individual needs. It's important to follow the recommended dosage on the product label or consult with a healthcare professional for personalized guidance.

How to Use: Cell Food is typically taken orally, either directly or mixed into water or juice. It's important to shake the bottle well before use and to store it according to the manufacturer's instructions.

Side Effects: Cell Food is generally considered safe for most people when used as directed. However, some individuals may experience mild digestive upset or allergic reactions to certain ingredients. It's essential to consult with a healthcare provider before starting any new supplement regimen, especially if you have underlying health conditions or are taking medications.

Chaparral:

Definition: Chaparral, scientifically known as Larrea tridentata, is a shrub native to the southwestern United States and northern Mexico. It has been used for centuries by Native American tribes for its medicinal properties and is commonly used in herbal medicine today.

Ingredients: Chaparral contains several bioactive compounds, including nordihydroguaiaretic acid (NDGA), flavonoids, lignans, and volatile oils. NDGA is believed to be the primary active compound responsible for many of chaparral's therapeutic effects.

How to Prepare: Chaparral can be prepared and consumed in various forms, including teas, tinctures, capsules, and topical preparations. To make tea, dried chaparral leaves are steeped in hot water for several minutes before being strained and consumed. Tinctures are prepared by steeping the herb in alcohol or vinegar to extract its active compounds.

Dosage: The appropriate dosage of chaparral can vary depending on the specific form and intended use. It's important to follow the recommended dosage on the product label or consult with a healthcare professional for personalized guidance.

How to Use: Chaparral tea or tincture is typically taken orally. It can also be applied topically to the skin for certain conditions. It's important to use chaparral products as directed and to discontinue use if any adverse effects occur.

Side Effects: Chaparral is generally considered safe for most people when used in moderate amounts. However, excessive intake or prolonged use may lead to liver toxicity or other adverse effects. It may also interact with certain medications or have adverse effects in individuals with certain health conditions. It's important to use chaparral under the guidance of a healthcare professional and to discontinue use if any adverse effects occur.

Cocolmeca:

Definition: Cocolmeca, also known as Smilax ornata or sarsaparilla, is a flowering vine native to Mexico and Central America. It has been used traditionally in Mexican and Central American folk medicine for its purported medicinal properties.

Ingredients: Cocolmeca contains various bioactive compounds, including saponins, flavonoids, and plant sterols. These compounds are believed to contribute to the herb's medicinal properties, including its potential as a diuretic, blood purifier, and anti-inflammatory agent.

How to Prepare: Cocolmeca is commonly prepared and consumed as an herbal tea or decoction. To make tea, dried cocolmeca roots or leaves are steeped in hot water for several minutes before being strained and consumed. Decoctions involve boiling the roots or leaves in water to extract their active compounds.

Dosage: The appropriate dosage of cocolmeca can vary depending on factors such as age, health status, and the specific preparation being used. It's important to follow the recommended dosage on the product label or consult with a qualified herbalist or healthcare professional for personalized guidance.

How to Use: Cocolmeca tea or decoction is typically taken orally. It can also be used topically for certain skin conditions. It's important to use cocolmeca products as directed and to discontinue use if any adverse effects occur.

Side Effects: Cocolmeca is generally considered safe for most people when used in moderate amounts. However, excessive intake may lead to digestive upset or other adverse effects. It may also interact with certain medications or have adverse effects in individuals with certain health conditions. It's important to use cocolmeca under the guidance of a healthcare professional and to discontinue use if any adverse effects occur.

Contribo:

Definition: Contribo, also known as Aristolochiatrilobata, is a vine native to the Caribbean and Central America. It has been used traditionally in folk medicine for various purposes, including as a remedy for digestive issues, inflammation, and pain relief.

Ingredients: Contribo contains several bioactive compounds, including aristolochic acids, flavonoids, and alkaloids. These compounds are believed to contribute to the herb's medicinal properties, including its potential as an anti-inflammatory and analgesic agent.

How to Prepare: Contribo is typically prepared and consumed as an herbal tea or decoction. To make tea, dried contribo leaves or stems are steeped in hot water for several minutes before being strained and consumed. Decoctions involve boiling the leaves or stems in water to extract their active compounds.

Dosage: The appropriate dosage of contribo can vary depending on factors such as age, health status, and the specific preparation being used. It's important to follow the recommended dosage on the product label or consult with a qualified herbalist or healthcare professional for personalized guidance.

How to Use: Contribo tea or decoction is typically taken orally. It's important to use contribo products as directed and to discontinue use if any adverse effects occur.

Side Effects: Contribo contains aristolochic acids, which have been associated with serious adverse effects, including kidney damage and cancer. Due to these safety concerns, the use of contribo is highly discouraged, and it's important to avoid products containing aristolochic acids. Individuals should seek alternative remedies for their health needs.

Guaco:

Definition: Guaco, also known as Mikania cordata or Mikania glomerata, is a medicinal plant native to Central and South America. It has a long history of use in traditional medicine for its potential therapeutic properties.

Ingredients: Guaco contains several bioactive compounds, including coumarins, flavonoids, tannins, and saponins. These compounds are believed to contribute to the herb's medicinal properties, including its potential as an expectorant, anti-inflammatory, and antispasmodic agent.

How to Prepare: Guaco is typically prepared and consumed as an herbal tea or infusion. To make tea, dried guaco leaves are steeped in hot water for several minutes before being strained and consumed.

Dosage: The appropriate dosage of guaco can vary depending on factors such as age, health status, and the specific preparation being used. It's important to follow the recommended dosage on the product label or consult with a qualified herbalist or healthcare professional for personalized guidance.

How to Use: Guaco tea is typically taken orally. It can be consumed on its own or mixed with honey or other herbal teas for added flavor.

Side Effects: Guaco is generally considered safe for most people when used in moderate amounts. However, some individuals may experience allergic reactions or digestive upset. It may also interact with certain medications or have adverse effects in individuals with certain health conditions. It's important to use guaco under the guidance of a healthcare professional and to discontinue use if any adverse effects occur.

Herban Iron:

Definition: Herban Iron is a dietary supplement designed to provide an easily absorbable form of iron to support healthy iron levels in the body. It's particularly beneficial for individuals with iron deficiency or anemia.

Ingredients: Herban Iron typically contains iron in the form of ferrous bisglycinate, which is a highly bioavailable and gentle form of iron that is less likely to cause digestive upset or constipation compared to other forms of iron. It may also contain other ingredients such as vitamin C to enhance iron absorption.

How to Prepare: Herban Iron is usually available in capsule or liquid form. Capsules are taken orally with water, while liquid forms may be mixed with water or juice before consumption. It's important to follow the recommended dosage on the product label.

Dosage: The appropriate dosage of Herban Iron depends on factors such as age, gender, and the severity of iron deficiency. It's important to consult with a healthcare professional to determine the correct dosage for individual needs.

How to Use: Herban Iron capsules are typically taken orally with water, while liquid forms may be mixed with water or juice before consumption. It's important to take Herban Iron as directed and to avoid taking it with dairy products, antacids, or other substances that may interfere with iron absorption.

Side Effects: While Herban Iron is generally considered safe for most people when used as directed, some individuals may experience mild side effects such as gastrointestinal discomfort or constipation. It's important to consult with a healthcare professional before starting any new supplement regimen, especially if you have underlying health conditions or are taking medications.

Hydrangea:

Definition: Hydrangea, scientifically known as Hydrangea arborescens, is a flowering shrub native to North America. It has been used traditionally in herbal medicine for its potential diuretic and anti-inflammatory properties.

Ingredients: Hydrangea contains several bioactive compounds, including saponins, flavonoids, and glycosides. These compounds are believed to contribute to the herb's medicinal properties, including its potential as a diuretic, kidney tonic, and anti-inflammatory agent.

How to Prepare: Hydrangea root is typically prepared and consumed as an herbal tea or tincture. To make tea, dried hydrangea root is steeped in hot water for several minutes before being strained and consumed. Tinctures are prepared by steeping the root in alcohol or vinegar to extract its active compounds.

Dosage: The appropriate dosage of hydrangea can vary depending on factors such as age, health status, and the specific preparation being used. It's important to follow the recommended dosage on the product label or consult with a qualified herbalist or healthcare professional for personalized guidance.

How to Use: Hydrangea tea or tincture is typically taken orally. It's important to use hydrangea products as directed and to discontinue use if any adverse effects occur.

Side Effects: Hydrangea is generally considered safe for most people when used in moderate amounts. However, some individuals may experience digestive upset or allergic reactions. It may also interact with certain medications or have adverse effects in individuals with certain health conditions. It's important to use hydrangea under the guidance of a healthcare professional and to discontinue use if any adverse effects occur.

Irish Moss:

Definition: Irish Moss, scientifically known as Chondrus crispus, is a species of red algae or seaweed native to the Atlantic coastlines of Europe and North America. It has been used for centuries in traditional Irish and Scottish cuisine, as well as in herbal medicine.

Ingredients: Irish Moss is rich in various nutrients, including iodine, sulfur compounds, vitamins (such as vitamin A, vitamin K, and vitamin B12), minerals (including calcium, magnesium, potassium, and sodium), and polysaccharides (such as carrageenan). These nutrients are believed to contribute to the herb's potential health benefits.

How to Prepare: Irish Moss is typically prepared by soaking it in water to rehydrate and soften it before use. It can be added to soups, stews, smoothies, desserts, and other dishes as a thickening agent or nutritional supplement.

Dosage: The appropriate dosage of Irish Moss can vary depending on factors such as age, health status, and the specific preparation being used. It's important to follow recipes or guidelines for culinary use and to consult with a healthcare professional for guidance on using Irish Moss as a dietary supplement.

How to Use: Irish Moss can be used in culinary applications to add thickness and nutritional value to dishes. It can also be consumed as a dietary supplement in the form of capsules, powders, or extracts.

Side Effects: Irish Moss is generally considered safe for most people when consumed in moderate amounts as part of a balanced diet. However, some individuals may be allergic to seaweed or carrageenan, a compound found in Irish Moss that is used as a food additive. It's important to discontinue use if any adverse effects occur and to consult with a healthcare professional if you have any concerns.

Irish Sea Moss:

Definition: Irish Sea Moss is a term often used interchangeably with Irish Moss, referring to the same species of red algae, Chondrus crispus. It's harvested from the rocky shores of the Atlantic coastlines of Europe and North America.

Ingredients: Irish Sea Moss shares the same nutritional profile as Irish Moss, containing iodine, vitamins, minerals, and polysaccharides. It's valued for its potential health benefits, including supporting thyroid function, boosting immune health, and promoting digestion.

How to Prepare: Irish Sea Moss is prepared in the same way as Irish Moss, by soaking it in water to rehydrate and soften it before use. It can be used in culinary applications or consumed as a dietary supplement.

Dosage: The dosage of Irish Sea Moss depends on the form and intended use. As a dietary supplement, it's important to follow the recommended dosage on the product label or consult with a healthcare professional for personalized guidance.

How to Use: Irish Sea Moss can be used in various culinary applications, including soups, smoothies, desserts, and sauces. It can also be consumed as a dietary supplement in the form of capsules, powders, or extracts.

Side Effects: Similar to Irish Moss, Irish Sea Moss is generally considered safe for most people when consumed in moderate amounts. However, individuals with seaweed allergies or sensitivities to carrageenan should exercise caution. It's important to discontinue use if any adverse effects occur and to consult with a healthcare professional if you have any concerns.

Lymphalin:

Definition: Lymphalin is a herbal supplement formulated to support lymphatic system health. The lymphatic system plays a crucial role in immune function and waste removal in the body, and Lymphalin is designed to promote its proper function.

Ingredients: Lymphalin typically contains a blend of herbs and botanical extracts known for their traditional use in supporting lymphatic system health. Common ingredients may include cleavers, red clover, echinacea, burdock root, and calendula, among others.

How to Prepare: Lymphalin is usually available in capsule or liquid form. Capsules are taken orally with water, while liquid forms may be mixed with water or juice before consumption. It's important to follow the recommended dosage on the product label.

Dosage: The appropriate dosage of Lymphalin can vary depending on the specific product and individual needs. It's important to follow the recommended dosage on the product label or consult with a healthcare professional for personalized guidance.

How to Use: Lymphalin capsules are typically taken orally with water, while liquid forms may be mixed with water or juice before consumption. It's often recommended to take Lymphalin on an empty stomach for optimal absorption.

Side Effects: Lymphalin is generally considered safe for most people when used as directed. However, some individuals may experience mild side effects such as gastrointestinal discomfort or allergic reactions to certain ingredients. It's important to consult with a healthcare provider before starting any new supplement regimen, especially if you have underlying health conditions or are taking medications.

Manjakani:

Definition: Manjakani, also known as Quercus infectoria or oak gall, is a natural substance derived from the oak tree. It has been used for centuries in traditional medicine for its potential health benefits, particularly for women's health and vaginal tightening.

Ingredients: Manjakani contains various bioactive compounds, including tannins, flavonoids, and gallic acid. These compounds are believed to contribute to the herb's medicinal properties, including its potential as an astringent and antiseptic agent.

How to Prepare: Manjakani is typically available in powder, capsule, or liquid extract form. It can be taken orally or used topically depending on the intended use. For vaginal tightening, manjakani may be applied topically as a gel or inserted into the vagina in capsule form.

Dosage: The appropriate dosage of manjakani can vary depending on factors such as age, health status, and the specific preparation being used. It's important to follow the recommended dosage on the product label or consult with a qualified herbalist or healthcare professional for personalized guidance.

How to Use: Manjakani can be taken orally or used topically depending on the intended use. It's important to use manjakani products as directed and to discontinue use if any adverse effects occur.

Side Effects: Manjakani is generally considered safe for most people when used in moderate amounts. However, some individuals may experience allergic reactions or skin irritation when used topically. It's important to use manjakani under the guidance of a healthcare professional and to discontinue use if any adverse effects occur.

Red Clover:

Definition: Red clover, scientifically known as Trifolium pratense, is a flowering plant belonging to the legume family. It's native to Europe, Western Asia, and Northwest Africa but has been naturalized in many other regions. Red clover has been used in traditional medicine for various purposes, including its potential to support women's health and menopausal symptoms.

Ingredients: Red clover contains several bioactive compounds, including isoflavones (such as genistein and daidzein), flavonoids, and phytoestrogens. These compounds are believed to contribute to the herb's medicinal properties, including its potential as a hormone-balancing agent and its ability to support cardiovascular health.

How to Prepare: Red clover is typically prepared and consumed as an herbal tea or tincture. To make tea, dried red clover flowers are steeped in hot water for several minutes before being strained and consumed. Tinctures are prepared by steeping the flowers in alcohol or vinegar to extract their active compounds.

Dosage: The appropriate dosage of red clover can vary depending on factors such as age, health status, and the specific preparation being used. It's important to follow the recommended dosage on the product label or consult with a qualified herbalist or healthcare professional for personalized guidance.

How to Use: Red clover tea or tincture is typically taken orally. It's important to use red clover products as directed and to discontinue use if any adverse effects occur.

Side Effects: Red clover is generally considered safe for most people when used in moderate amounts. However, some individuals may experience allergic reactions or digestive upset. It may also interact with certain medications or have adverse effects in individuals with certain health conditions. It's important to use red clover under the guidance of a healthcare professional and to discontinue use if any adverse effects occur.

Rhubarb:

Definition: Rhubarb, scientifically known as Rheum rhabarbarum, is a perennial plant cultivated for its edible stalks. While primarily used in culinary applications, rhubarb has also been utilized in traditional medicine for its potential health benefits, particularly for digestive health.

Ingredients: Rhubarb stalks contain various bioactive compounds, including anthraquinones (such as emodin and rhein), fiber, vitamins (such as vitamin K), and minerals (including calcium and potassium). These compounds are believed to contribute to the herb's medicinal properties, including its potential as a laxative and digestive aid.

How to Prepare: Rhubarb stalks are typically cooked before consumption, as the raw stalks are very tart and can be unpleasant to eat. They are often used in pies, crisps, jams, sauces, and other desserts, as well as in savory dishes. Rhubarb can also be used to make compotes, jams, and preserves.

Dosage: There is no specific dosage for rhubarb in culinary applications, as it is used as a food rather than a medicinal herb. However, when used for its potential laxative effects, it's important to consume rhubarb in moderation to avoid gastrointestinal upset.

How to Use: Rhubarb stalks can be chopped and cooked in various dishes, including pies, sauces, and jams. It's important to remove and discard the leaves, as they contain toxic compounds. When using rhubarb for its potential laxative effects, it's typically consumed as part of a cooked dish or in the form of a rhubarb-based herbal remedy.

Side Effects: Rhubarb stalks are generally safe for most people when consumed in moderate amounts as part of a balanced diet. However, excessive intake may lead to digestive upset or adverse effects due to the presence of oxalic acid, which can bind to calcium and form kidney stones in susceptible individuals. It's important to use rhubarb in moderation and to consult with a healthcare professional if you have any concerns or underlying health conditions.

Tila:

Definition: Tila, also known as linden flower or lime blossom, refers to the flowers of the Tilia genus, primarily Tilia europaea and Tilia cordata. These trees are native to Europe, but they are also cultivated in other regions for their fragrant and medicinal flowers.

Ingredients: Tila flowers contain various bioactive compounds, including flavonoids, phenolic acids, and volatile oils. These compounds are believed to contribute to the herb's medicinal properties, including its potential as a mild sedative, anxiolytic, and anti-inflammatory agent.

How to Prepare: Tila flowers are typically prepared and consumed as an herbal tea or infusion. To make tea, dried tila flowers are steeped in hot water for several minutes before being strained and consumed.

Dosage: The appropriate dosage of tila can vary depending on factors such as age, health status, and the specific preparation being used. It's important to follow the recommended dosage on the product label or consult with a qualified herbalist or healthcare professional for personalized guidance.

How to Use: Tila tea is typically taken orally. It's often consumed in the evening as a calming bedtime beverage or during times of stress or anxiety. It's important to use tila products as directed and to discontinue use if any adverse effects occur.

Side Effects: Tila is generally considered safe for most people when used in moderate amounts. However, some individuals may experience allergic reactions or digestive upset. It may also interact with certain medications or have adverse effects in individuals with certain health conditions. It's important to use tila under the guidance of a healthcare professional and to discontinue use if any adverse effects occur.

Yellowdock Root:

Definition: Yellowdock root, scientifically known as Rumex crispus, is the root of a perennial flowering plant native to Europe and western Asia, also found in North America. It has a long history of use in traditional medicine, particularly among Indigenous peoples, for its potential health benefits.

Ingredients: Yellowdock root contains various bioactive compounds, including anthraquinone glycosides (such as emodin and chrysophanol), tannins, and vitamins (including vitamin A and vitamin C). These compounds are believed to contribute to the herb's medicinal properties, including its potential as a laxative, blood cleanser, and liver tonic.

How to Prepare: Yellowdock root is typically prepared and consumed as an herbal tea, tincture, or capsule. To make tea, dried yellowdock root is steeped in hot water for several minutes before being strained and consumed. Tinctures are prepared by steeping the root in alcohol or vinegar to extract its active compounds.

Dosage: The appropriate dosage of yellowdock root can vary depending on factors such as age, health status, and the specific preparation being used. It's important to follow the recommended dosage on the product label or consult with a qualified herbalist or healthcare professional for personalized guidance.

How to Use: Yellowdock root tea, tincture, or capsules are typically taken orally. It's often consumed to support digestion, promote bowel regularity, and cleanse the blood. It's important to use yellowdock root products as directed and to discontinue use if any adverse effects occur.

Side Effects: Yellowdock root is generally considered safe for most people when used in moderate amounts. However, some individuals may experience mild side effects such as gastrointestinal upset or allergic reactions. It may also interact with certain medications or have adverse effects in individuals with certain health conditions. It's important to use yellowdock root under the guidance of a healthcare professional and to discontinue use if any adverse effects occur.

Dandelion Root:

Definition: Dandelion, scientifically known as Taraxacum officinale, is a common flowering plant found worldwide. While often considered a pesky weed, dandelion has a long history of use in traditional medicine for its various health benefits.

Ingredients: Dandelion root contains several bioactive compounds, including sesquiterpene lactones, triterpenes, flavonoids, and polysaccharides. These compounds are believed to contribute to the herb's medicinal properties, including its potential as a diuretic, digestive aid, and liver tonic.

How to Prepare: Dandelion root can be prepared and consumed in various forms, including teas, tinctures, capsules, and extracts. To make tea, dried dandelion root is steeped in hot water for several minutes before being strained and consumed. Tinctures are prepared by steeping the root in alcohol or vinegar to extract its active compounds.

Dosage: The appropriate dosage of dandelion root can vary depending on factors such as age, health status, and the specific preparation being used. It's important to follow the recommended dosage on the product label or consult with a qualified herbalist or healthcare professional for personalized guidance.

How to Use: Dandelion root tea, tincture, or capsules are typically taken orally. It's important to use dandelion root products as directed and to discontinue use if any adverse effects occur.

Side Effects: Dandelion root is generally considered safe for most people when used in moderate amounts. However, some individuals may experience allergic reactions or digestive upset. It may also interact with certain medications or have adverse effects in individuals with certain health conditions. It's important to use dandelion root under the guidance of a healthcare professional and to discontinue use if any adverse effects occur.

Green Food Plus:

Definition: Green Food Plus is a dietary supplement formulated to provide a concentrated source of nutrients derived from various green plants. It's designed to support overall health and well-being by delivering essential vitamins, minerals, antioxidants, and phytonutrients.

Ingredients: Green Food Plus typically contains a blend of powdered green vegetables, grasses, algae, and other plant-based ingredients. Common ingredients may include wheatgrass, barley grass, spirulina, chlorella, alfalfa, kale, spinach, and broccoli, among others.

How to Prepare: Green Food Plus is usually available in powder form and can be mixed with water, juice, or smoothies. It's important to follow the recommended dosage on the product label and to consume it as part of a balanced diet.

Dosage: The appropriate dosage of Green Food Plus can vary depending on the specific product and individual needs. It's important to follow the recommended dosage on the product label or consult with a healthcare professional for personalized guidance.

How to Use: Green Food Plus powder is typically mixed with water, juice, or smoothies and consumed orally. It's often taken once or twice daily, preferably with meals, to maximize nutrient absorption.

Side Effects: Green Food Plus is generally considered safe for most people when used as directed. However, some individuals may experience digestive upset or allergic reactions to certain ingredients. It's important to consult with a healthcare provider before starting any new supplement regimen, especially if you have underlying health conditions or are taking medications.

THE END